Exercises

FOR

Gentlemen

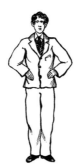

Exercises
FOR
Gentlemen

50 Exercises
TO DO WITH YOUR
Suit on

ALFRED B. OLSEN M.D. AND
M. ELLSWORTH OLSEN, M.A.

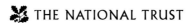

THE NATIONAL TRUST

ISBN-13: 978-1-905400-77-5

A CIP catalogue record for this book is available from
the British Library.

This book was conceived, designed, and produced by

Ivy Press
The Old Candlemakers,
West Street, Lewes,
East Sussex, BN7 2NZ
www.ivy-group.co.uk

Creative Director Peter Bridgewater
Publisher Jason Hook
Editorial Director Caroline Earle
Project Editor James Thomas
Art Director Clare Harris
Design JC Lanaway
Additional Illustrations Coral Mula

Printed in China

10 9 8 7 6 5 4 3 2 1

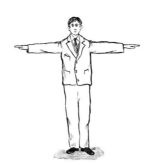

CONTENTS

" How, then, shall we cultivate that condition of the body which will enable it most perfectly to reflect the beauty of the soul within? "

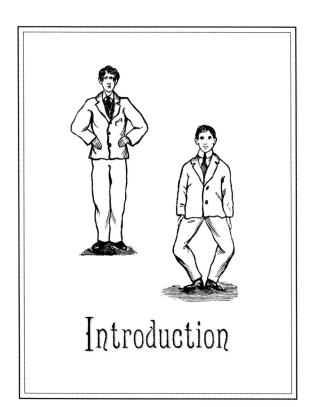

Introduction

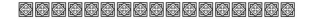

GUIDING PRINCIPLES

A few words may be said in regard to the purpose of this book. It aims to be a sort of text-book in health culture from which any individual can obtain the necessary guidance in a systematic course of physical improvement. It would fain inspire in its readers respect for their bodies as the Creator's chief handiwork, and a determination not to abuse them in any way, but rather to develop their powers to the utmost. It would stimulate in every young man a noble ambition to arrive at complete physical realisation, to cultivate not bigness so much as health of muscle and soundness of all organs of the body, to abhor stimulants and narcotics, to shun bad habits and fashionable dissipation, and to count it a joy to render hearty obedience to every natural law. With such ideals in the home, health would indeed spring forth speedily, and the clear, rosy cheeks, the sparkling eyes, the elastic step, and alert, vigorous carriage that we all so much admire would be very much more in evidence.

If one guiding principle be sought for upon which life can be remodelled, we commend the "Simple Life." Get back to nature. This does not mean to savagery; it does not involve renouncing all the conveniences of civilisation; but it does mean to turn one's back on the soul-deadening artificialities and machine methods, and the mad, feverish rush after wealth which are eating into the very heart of present-day society. It means to cultivate simple, natural habits, and take one's recreations as far as possible out-of-doors.

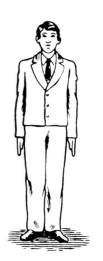

The toiler in our large cities can live the simple life, or at least a modified version of it. He may be obliged to work in the city when he would rather be in the country; but his habits will be simple, his needs few and easily supplied; and when the hours of recreation come, they will not find him in a stuffy theatre or music hall, but out under the open heavens, drinking in the life-giving oxygen, and gathering strength for the task of the morrow. Circumstances may imprison him for a time, even as a cage imprisons the bird, but once the door is open, he is away to the fields and the woods which are his natural home.

Such in spirit is the simple life. That it is also a healthful and happy life. When it becomes even so much as an aspiration in any home an important step has been taken towards higher things.

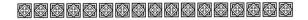

BEAUTY CULTURE

Emerson tells us: "The fountain of beauty is the heart, and every generous thought illustrates the walls of your chamber."

"Then it doesn't matter how we treat our bodies," someone may say, "if beauty is a spiritual thing." Yes, it matters a great deal, for if the glass is dingy and coated over with filth, then the image it conveys will be a blurred one. Thus many a beautiful and cultured mind must, owing to the neglect of beauty culture of the right kind, look forth through a body disfigured by disease.

How, then, shall we cultivate that condition of the body which will enable it most perfectly to reflect the beauty of the soul within? This is surely no small, insignificant matter, but one in which everybody must be interested.

No True Beauty Without Health.

First, there can be no true beauty without health. The clear sparkling eyes, the rosy cheeks, the transparent skin – are not all these so many signals that Nature hangs out to show that all is well within? Then, whatever is injurious to the health of the body must also spoil its beauty; and, on the other hand, that which makes for health and long life, likewise must make for beauty.

Exercise as a Beautifier.

Daily exercise out-of-doors is a wonderful beautifier. It improves the circulation, gives tone to the nerves, rounds out the muscles, and imparts stay and stamina to the system.

Brisk walking with chest well expanded, shoulders back, and arms hanging naturally at the sides, is the best all-round exercise. Riding, cycling, tennis, croquet, and golf are all very good taken in moderation. Working in the garden is also excellent provided care is taken to avoid an undue amount of stooping, which contracts the chest.

A graceful carriage, which is one of the primary elements of beauty, may be cultivated by practising the light gymnastics given in the following chapters on physical development. Swimming is also a capital exercise for those who wish to acquire a degree of ease and grace of movement.

Deep breathing, practised night and morning, will do wonders in the way of broadening and deepening the chest, and filling up the unsightly hollows of the neck and chest.

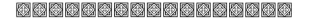

PHYSICAL DEVELOPMENT

I t was a saying of Herbert Spencer that the first essential to success in life is "a good animal." Certainly the man who is blessed with firm, elastic muscles, an erect carriage, and a state of general physical fitness, possesses a formidable equipment for the battle of life. His superiority to those less richly endowed physically will show itself in a great many ways. Exercise in moderation and the symmetrical development of the body are of the greatest value in maintaining a state of health and vital efficiency. Sufficient use of the muscles to keep them in good condition is favourable to the accomplishment of the best mental work *(Fig. 1)*.

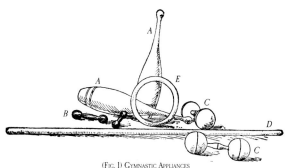

(FIG. 1) GYMNASTIC APPLIANCES
a. Indian Clubs; b. Iron dumb-bells; c. Wooden dumb-bells; d. Wand; e. Ring

Benefits of Exercise.

Firstly, it greatly aids digestion, thus improving the nutrition of all organs, including the brain.

Secondly, it quickens breathing, both in the lungs and in the tissues.

Thirdly, it stimulates the circulation, sending the purified blood bounding through the arteries and into the minute capillaries throughout the entire body.

Fourthly, a good condition of muscular fitness usually brings sound, refreshing sleep, and a well-balanced nervous system.

Fifthly, and finally, it contributes to that calm self-possession, that well-balanced air, that combination of strength and gentleness, which is so attractive in either sex.

The Meaning of Flabby Muscles.

There are, of course, exceptions, but as a general rule, flabby muscles may be taken to denote a general mental, if not moral, flabbiness; while the training of the muscles, kept within the proper limits, wonderfully enlivens the spirits and the general tone of a person, mentally as well as physically. Study the lives of the men who have left their mark in the history of the world, and, though they may differ in many respects, you will find that they were mostly alike in possessing a certain firmness of muscular texture, and the ability to endure severe strain, physical and mental.

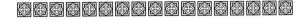

THE BENEFITS OF EXERCISE

In this book we shall endeavour to give busy men some practical instruction in physical culture of a character suited to their requirements. We shall not aim to make Sandows[1] of them, but rather show each how to improve physique, strengthen the weak organs, make firm the flabby muscles, increase chest capacity, reduce undue fullness at the waist, square the shoulders, round out the arms, improve leg development, and, in short, make a more graceful, strong, and symmetrical man.

All this can be done by means of the following very carefully arranged exercises, provided they are faithfully taken. Fifteen minutes daily is all that is absolutely required, though ten minutes in the morning and again in the evening will be even more satisfactory; and persons who are especially deficient would do well to make it fifteen.

1. Sandow was the Arnie of his day

Precautions.

Just a few general precautions before giving the exercises. First and foremost, *put your whole heart into everything you do*. When taking arm exercises, let your mind power be concentrated on your arms – not painfully, but cheerfully and earnestly. When taking breathing exercises, do them also with a will and heartily, fixing the attention on the lungs and the muscles of respiration.

Take the exercises when you are feeling best. Never take them when physically weary. Endeavour at the same time to be regular, so that a certain hour each day will always find you busily engaged in this scientific muscle culture.

Have the room well ventilated, and, if possible, bright and sunny. Exercise always in a cheerful mood. Determine to enjoy the process of developing your muscles, for, as the poet well puts it—

"No profit grows where is no pleasure ta'en."

In the interests of conciseness, we give here, in their proper order, some of the fundamental positions which will be used in their various combinations. The reader who expects to take up physical culture in earnest will do well to familiarise himself with the terms applied to these positions.

✳ ✳ ✳ ✳ ✳

" If the directions have been carefully followed,

the position will be one of erectness, dignity,

and grace, and pleasing to behold "

✳ ✳ ✳ ✳ ✳

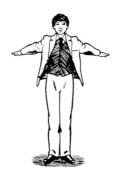

Chapter 1

Standing
Exercises

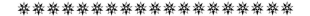

SIMPLE STANDING EXERCISES

Exercise 1: Standing, Primary Position.

To take the correct standing position, stand with the back to a door or wall. The heels should touch each other, and the feet must form a right angle. The heels, hips, back, and head should touch the wall, and the arms hang loosely.

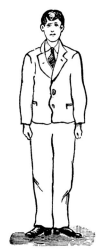

(FIG. 2) STANDING, PRIMARY POSITION

While maintaining the erect position, bend the head backwards as far as possible. This pushes the chest forward and upward, and separates the back from the wall. While maintaining this position raise the head, keeping the chin well in. Only the heels and hips now touch the wall, and the centre of gravity passes through the balls of the feet *(Fig. 2)*. Test the position by raising the heels. If this can be done without throwing the body forward, the position is correct.

If the directions have been carefully followed, the position will be one of erectness, dignity, and grace, and pleasing to behold. More, it gives spring and elasticity to the step, and in walking minimises jarring of the spine.

Such is the proper standing position for man. It gives freedom of action to the lungs and all the other organs of the body. At first the position will be tiring, if one is not accustomed to standing erect, and considerable practice may be necessary in order to make it a natural habit.

COMPOUND STANDING POSITIONS

We shall now give a few compound standing positions which will be used in taking some of the movements to be described later. In all cases the correct standing position (see Exercise 1) is the basis of the exercise, the only difference being the position of the limbs.

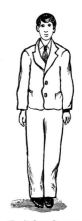

(Fig. 3) Close Standing

Exercise 2: Close Standing.
The feet are held close together, touching at the balls as well as at the heels *(Fig. 3)*.

Exercise 3: Toe-Standing.
Identical with correct standing, except that the heels are raised from the ground about two or three inches *(Fig. 4)*.

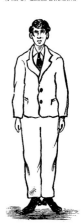

(Fig. 4) Toe-Standing

Exercise 4: Knee-Bend-Standing.

Similar to Exercise 1, except that the knees are bent to a right angle *(Fig. 5)*.

Exercise 5: Wing-Standing.

Take the standing position (see Exercise 1), and then let the hands rest on the hips, with thumbs behind the fingers in front. The elbows form right angles, and are in the same plane as the trunk. Avoid bending the wrists. The arm and hand should form a straight line from the elbow to the tip of the index finger *(Fig. 6)*.

Exercise 6: Bend-Standing.

This is the same as Exercise 1, with the exception of the arms, which are close to the body, while the forearms are bent upward, the fingers resting on the shoulders *(Fig. 7)*.

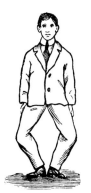
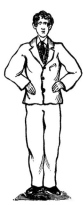
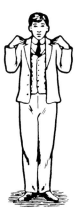

(Fig. 5) Knee-Bend-Standing   (Fig. 6) Wing-Standing   (Fig. 7) Bend-Standing

Exercise 7: Heave-Standing.

In this position the upper arms are extended outwards, forming right angles with the trunk. The fore-arms are extended upward from the elbows with palms facing, and forming right angles with the upper arms. Both arms are in the same plane as the trunk *(Fig. 8)*.

Exercise 8: Rest-Standing.

The hands are placed behind the neck with palms forward and fingers touching. The elbows should be well back, in the same plane as the trunk. There is always the tendency to bend the head forward, which should be guarded against. It is an excellent position for expanding the chest *(Fig. 9)*.

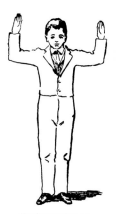

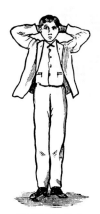

(Fig. 8) Heave-Standing   (Fig. 9) Rest-Standing

Exercise 9: Stretch-Standing.

This identical with Exercise 1, except that the arms are extended straight upward with the palms facing each other *(Fig. 10)*.

Exercise 10: Yard-Standing.

Take a correct standing position, as described in Exercise 1, and then raise the arms outward to a level with the shoulders, keeping the fingers closed and the palms turned down *(Fig. 11)*.

These positions may be used in taking most of the following movements and exercises. It is important to take each initial position accurately as described in order to derive the full benefit from the exercise.

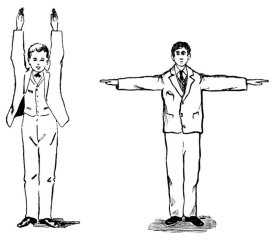

(Fig. 10) Stretch-Standing   (Fig. 11) Yard-Standing

" Exercise contributes to that calm self-possession, that well-balanced air, that combination of strength and gentleness, which is so attractive in either sex "

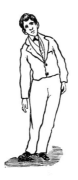

Chapter 2

Head & Trunk
Exercises

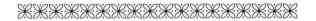

Simple Head & Trunk Exercises

Head Movements.

We shall only describe two movements of the head – bending and twisting. Combined with the correct standing position, these will be ample to ensure the health and mobility of the upper spine and neck.

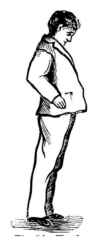

(Fig. 12)
Wing-Standing, Head-Bending

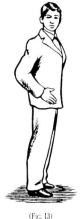

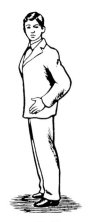

(Fig. 13)
Wing-Standing, Head-Twisting I

(Fig. 14)
Wing-Standing, Head-Twisting II

Exercise 11: Wing-Standing, Head-Bending & Head-Twisting.

While maintaining the correct standing position, bend the head forward as far as possible *(Fig. 12)*.

Then bend the head to the right, left, and backward. Repeat each flexion three to twelve times.

Turn the head slowly to the right as far as possible *(Fig. 13)*, and replace.

Then to the left *(Fig. 14)*. Turn the head alternately right and left. Repeat each three to twelve times.

TRUNK MOVEMENTS

Movements of the trunk should be taken rather slowly and deliberately as a rule. In this way the greatest benefit will be derived.

Exercise 12: Wing-Standing,
Trunk-Bending.

Forward.

Bend the trunk forward from the hips, keeping a strong inward curve in the back *(Fig. 15)*.

Repeat three to twelve times.

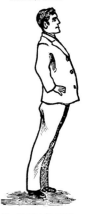

(Fig. 15)
WING-STANDING, TRUNK-
BENDING, FORWARD

Backward.

This movement is somewhat difficult, and due care should be taken not to strain the back. At best, the backward bending will be comparatively slight; nevertheless, the movement is a vigorous one if taken properly.

Take the wing-standing position, and then bend the trunk backward, keeping the relative position of the head the same as in standing. If correctly done, the body will form a bow from heel to head *(Fig. 16)*.

Repeat two to six times.

(Fig. 16) WING-STANDING,
TRUNK-BENDING, BACKWARD

Exercise 13: Standing, Trunk-Bending, Sideward.

Take the standing position and bend the trunk to the right as far as possible. Do not allow the head to drop to the side.

Repeat three to twelve times *(Fig. 17)*.

Do likewise to the left side.

Exercise 14: Wing-Standing, Trunk-Twisting.

Twist the trunk slowly to the left as far as possible, without straining, and then return to position. See that the twisting is in the spinal column above the hips, the latter remaining in the usual position during the movement *(Fig. 18)*.

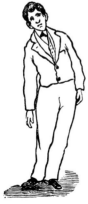

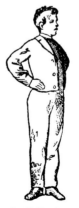

(Fig. 17) Wing-Standing, Trunk-Bending, Sideward

(Fig. 18) Wing-Standing, Trunk-Twisting

" The trunk should be erect, the chest well forward, the head erect, chin in, and there should be a strong upward stance of the spine "

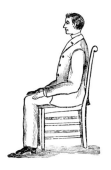

Chapter 3

Sitting, Walking, Climbing & Running

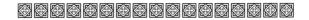

MAINTAINING
CORRECT POSTURE

Whether sitting, walking, climbing or running one should aim to maintain a correct, upright posture, which will ensure both elegance and symmetry.

CORRECT SITTING

Exercise 15: Sitting, Primary Position.

The chair or stool should be of such height as to allow the feet to rest comfortably on the floor. The trunk

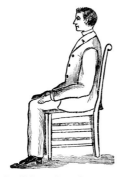

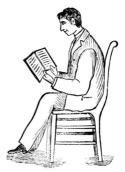

(FIG. 19) SITTING, PRIMARY POSITION   (FIG. 20) INCORRECT SITTING

should be erect, the chest well forward, the head erect, chin in, and there should be a strong upward stance of the spine *(Fig. 19)*.

Sitting so that the spine is arched forward is a pernicious habit that interferes with proper respiration *(Fig. 20)*. It should be avoided.

The proper way to sit down is to bend the knees and hips, keeping the trunk erect.

WALKING

Exercise 16: Walking.

Take the correct standing position, and constantly maintain the erect posture of the trunk. Bend the body forward from the hips, and step forward lightly, letting the weight of the body fall forward on the balls of the feet. The arms may swing at the sides.

Walking is sometimes described as an intermittent falling forward, with a foot thrust forward just in time to prevent falling *(Fig. 21)*.

There should be very little side sway of the body, and the step should be brisk and certain. If the position is correct, there will be a feeling of ease and elasticity that the old stooping gait could never give.

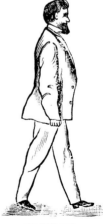

(FIG. 21) WALKING

33

CLIMBING EXERCISES

Exercise 17: Climbing Stairs.

Most people make the mistake of stooping forward when going up stairs. Such an unnatural position makes the climbing difficult and laborious *(Fig. 22)*. Walk up stairs as you would on the level, and you will be able to accomplish with comparative ease what is usually considered to be a wearisome task. A very slight forward bend of the trunk at the hip joints is all that is required to maintain proper equilibrium *(Fig. 23)*.

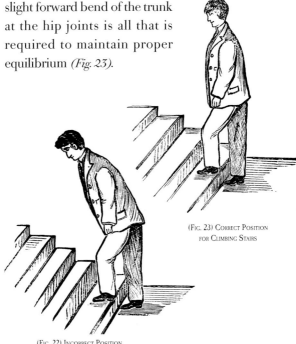

(FIG. 23) CORRECT POSITION
FOR CLIMBING STAIRS

(FIG. 22) INCORRECT POSITION
FOR CLIMBING STAIRS

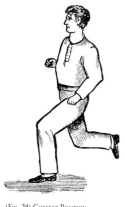

(Fig. 24) Correct Position
for Running

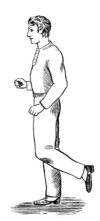

(Fig. 25) Incorrect Position
for Running

RUNNING EXERCISES

Exercise 18: Running.

The initial position is correct standing (Exercise 1) with the chest well forward. The heels scarcely touch the ground, and, at each stride, both feet are off the ground for a moment. The elbows are bent, and the hands loosely clenched. The movement is really a rapid falling forward, the lower limbs coming forward to support the body and preventing a fall *(Figs. 24 and 25)*.

✻ ✻ ✻ ✻ ✻

" When taking breathing exercises, do them
with a will and heartily, fixing the attention on the
lungs and the muscles of respiration "

✻ ✻ ✻ ✻ ✻

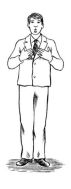

Chapter 4

Breathing
Exercises

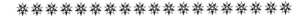

SIMPLE BREATHING EXERCISES

Before describing the movements of the trunk and other parts of the body, we will give a few simple breathing exercises. They may be taken lying, sitting, or standing, according to the requirements of the individual case. Also, ensure that there is plenty of fresh air to breathe.

Exercise 19: Deep Breathing.
Take the standing position (Exercise 1) and inhale slowly, filling the lungs to their utmost capacity. Then breathe out slowly. To breathe properly, there must be free action of the chest and abdominal muscles. During inspiration there should be an increase in the three diameters of the chest, antero-posterior, lateral, and vertical, shown in the diagram (Fig. 26).

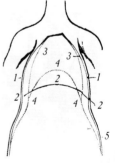

(Fig. 26) Diagram Showing Changes in the Chest Cavity During Respiration
1,2 Straight lines, showing expanded chest; 3,4, Dotted lines, showing contracted chest after expiration.

In expiration these same diameters are all diminished in size.

Constriction of any sort must be avoided. In breathing, use both chest and the abdominal muscles. This is properly known as costo-abdominal breathing. Always breathe through the nose. Repeat the process three to twelve times.

Exercise 20: Deep Breathing, Holding the Breath.

Inhale the air as directed in Exercise 19, and, when the lungs are full, hold the breath for half a minute or longer, and then empty the lungs. Repeat three to twelve times.

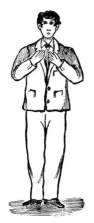

Exercise 21: Deep Breathing with Percussion.

This is the same as Exercise 20, except that, while holding the breath, the hands alternately strike the chest gently. Repeat three to twelve times *(Fig. 27)*.

(Fig. 27) Deep Breathing with Percussion

Exercise 22: Deep Breathing, Sounding "Ah!"

This is similar to Exercise 19, but, in exhaling, the sound "ah" is made distinctly and clearly as long as possible.

Repeat three to twelve times *(Fig. 28)*.

Exercise 23: Explosive Breathing.

Inhale slowly to your full capacity, and then breathe out quickly *(Fig. 29)*. This exercise may be reversed, inhaling quickly, and breathing out slowly, or the lungs may be filled and emptied rapidly. Repeat two to six times. These breathing exercises may be combined with many of the following movements, especially the raising of the arms upward above the head or extending them backward, and with the head movements *(see page 26)*.

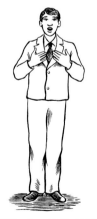
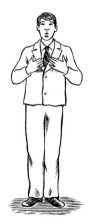

(Fig. 28) Deep Breathing, Sounding "Ah!"　　　(Fig. 29) Explosive Breathing

Exercise 24: Deep Breathing, Arms-Raising.

Backward.

Stand with the arms at the sides. While inhaling the air, gradually raise the arms backward. This movement serves to push the chest forward and upward, and thus favours respiration.

Repeat two to six times.

Forward, Upward.

While breathing in, slowly raise the extended arms forward and upward until directly above the head. The arms should be kept parallel and extended, and the palms facing. The air is exhaled while the arms are slowly returned to position.

This exercise should be taken with deliberation. An effort should be made to reach as far as possible with the fingers while executing the movement.

Repeat two to six times.

" Let your mind power be
concentrated on your arms – not
painfully, but cheerfully and earnestly "

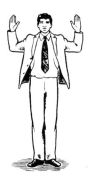

Chapter 5

Arm, Shoulder & Finger Exercises

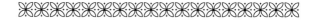

SIMPLE ARM, SHOULDER & FINGER EXERCISES

Arm and Finger Movements.

These are some of the most interesting and valuable exercises. Those involving the shoulders serve to strengthen the chest as well as the arms, and thus improve breathing. Unless otherwise directed, do them with vim and alacrity.

Exercise 25: Arm-Raising.

Forward.

Raise the right arm forward to a level with the shoulder, keeping it straight and well extended, and ensuring that the palm is turned inward.

Do likewise with the left arm.

Alternate, first the right arm and then the left.

Raise both arms together *(Fig. 30)*.

Repeat each movement three to twelve times.

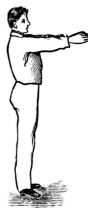

(FIG. 30)
ARM-RAISING, FORWARD

44

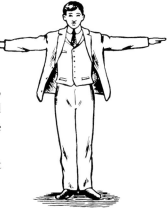

Outward.

This is similar to Exercise 25, except the arms are raised sideways instead of forward. The palms should face downward.

Repeat each movement three to twelve times *(Fig. 31)*.

(FIG. 31)
ARM-RAISING, OUTWARD

Exercise 26: Standing, Arm-Raising, Backward.

This movement, too, is similar to Exercise 25, but in this case the arms are raised and extended backward as far as possible without straining. The palms should face each other.

First raise the right arm backward, and then the left.

Alternate right and left.

Raise both arms together.

Repeat each movement three to twelve times *(Fig. 32)*.

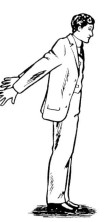

(FIG. 32) STANDING, ARM-RAISING, BACKWARD

Exercise 27: Standing, Arm-Stretching.
Standing in the usual position, with arms at the side, reach downward with both arms as far as possible *(Fig. 33)*.

With arms extended sideways on a level with the shoulders, reach outward as far as possible *(Fig. 34)*.

Extend the arms forward on a level with the shoulders, and reach forward as far as possible *(Fig. 35)*.

Now extend the arms upward, as in "stretch-standing" (Exercise 9), and reach upward *(Fig. 36)*.

Repeat each movement between two and six times.

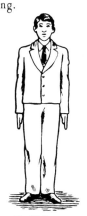

(Fig. 33) STANDING, ARM-STRETCHING

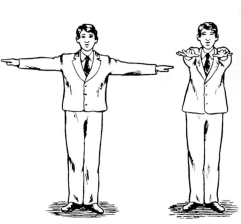

(Fig. 34) STANDING, ARM-STRETCHING, OUTWARD

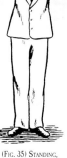

(Fig. 35) STANDING, ARM-STRETCHING, FORWARD

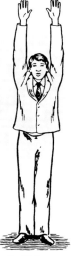

(Fig. 36) STANDING, ARM-STRETCHING, UPWARD

Exercise 28: Bend-Standing, Arm-Extending.
Downward.

For the initial position, see *Fig 37.*

Next, extend the right arm downward as far as possible *(Fig. 38)*, with the palm turned inward; likewise the left arm *(Fig. 39)*; then each alternately; and lastly both together *(Fig. 40)*.

Repeat each movement two to six times.

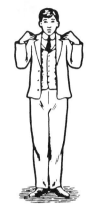

(Fig. 37) Bend-Standing, Arm-Extending, Downward I

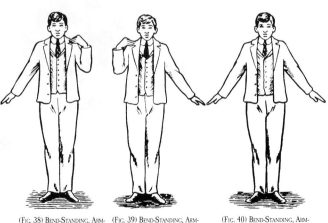

(Fig. 38) Bend-Standing, Arm-Extending, Downward II

(Fig. 39) Bend-Standing, Arm-Extending, Downward III

(Fig. 40) Bend-Standing, Arm-Extending, Downward IV

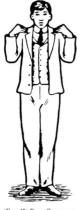

(FIG. 41) BEND-STANDING,
ARM-EXTENDING, FORWARD I

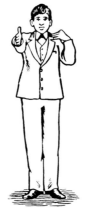

(FIG. 42) BEND-STANDING,
ARM-EXTENDING, FORWARD II

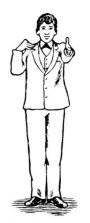

(FIG. 43) BEND-STANDING,
ARM-EXTENDING, FORWARD III

Forward.

This is the same as Exercise 28, except that the arms are extended forward, with palms facing each other *(Figs. 41 to 44)*.

Repeat each movement two to six times.

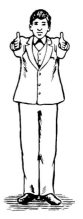

(FIG. 44) BEND-STANDING,
ARM-EXTENDING, FORWARD IV

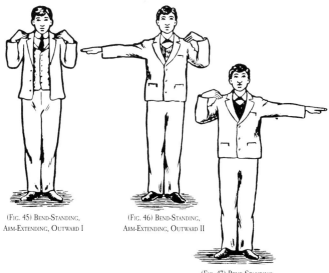

(Fig. 45) Bend-Standing,
Arm-Extending, Outward I

(Fig. 46) Bend-Standing,
Arm-Extending, Outward II

(Fig. 47) Bend-Standing,
Arm-Extending, Outward III

Outward.

In this exercise the arms are
extended outwards from
the side of the body, with
palms turned downward;
first the right arm, then the left,
then alternately, and lastly both
together *(Figs. 45 to 48)*.

Repeat each movement two to
six times.

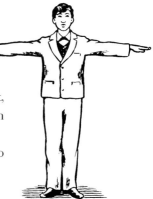

(Fig. 48) Bend-Standing,
Arm-Extending, Outward IV

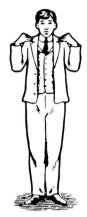

*Up*ward.

Starting in the position shown in *Fig. 49*, extend the arms straight upward, with palms facing each other, in the order described for "Bend-standing, arm-extending outward" *(Figs. 50 to 52)*.

Repeat each movement two to six times.

(FIG. 49) BEND-STANDING, ARM-EXTENDING, UPWARD I

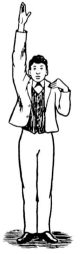

(FIG. 50) BEND-STANDING, ARM-EXTENDING, UPWARD II

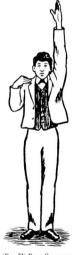

(FIG. 51) BEND-STANDING, ARM-EXTENDING, UPWARD III

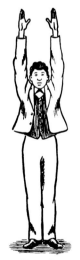

(FIG. 52) BEND-STANDING, ARM-EXTENDING, UPWARD IV

Exercise 29:
Heave-Standing,
Arm-Bending, Inward.

For the initial position, see Exercise 7. Bend the fore-arms inwards, touching the shoulders with the fingers.

Repeat three to twelve times.

Exercise 30: Heave-Standing, Arm-Extending.

Extend the arms outward with the palms turned upward, making sure to keep them at a level with the shoulders *(Fig. 53)*.

Repeat three to twelve times.

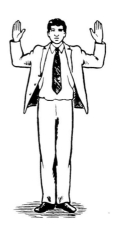

(FIG. 53) HEAVE-STANDING, ARM-EXTENDING

Exercise 31: Heave-Standing, Fore-Arm Rotating, Forward.

Rotate the fore-arms forward to a level with the shoulders *(Fig. 54)*.

Repeat three to twelve times.

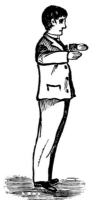

(FIG. 54) HEAVE-STANDING, FORE-ARM ROTATING, FORWARD

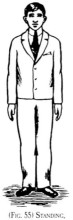

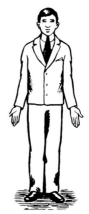

(FIG. 55) STANDING,
ARM-TWISTING &
ARM ROTATING I

(FIG. 56) STANDING,
ARM-TWISTING &
ARM ROTATING II

Exercise 32: Standing, Arm-Twisting & Arm Rotating.

With the arms hanging at the sides, twist both outward. The arms must be kept at full extension during the twisting. Then twist inward, and lastly alternate the movements. Repeat each movement three to twelve times.

Bring the right arm forward, upward, and backward, describing as large a circle as possible with the pointed fingers. Keep the elbow well extended. Repeat two to six times.

Now reverse the movement, and again repeat two to six times.

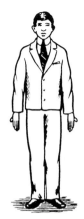

Rotate the left arm in a similar manner to the right.

Now rotate both arms together, first in one direction, and then in the other *(Figs. 55 to 57)*. Repeat each two to six times.

Exercise 33: Standing, Swimming. Take the correct standing position and bend the arms inward with palms turned down and fingers touching. The elbows should be on a level with the shoulders *(Fig. 58)*.

(FIG. 57) STANDING, ARM-TWISTING & ARM ROTATING III

Now extend both arms forward with palms turned outward, then back as far as possible, then return to the initial position.

Execute the movements with precision and vim.

Throughout these different positions, the arms should always be kept well extended, and at the same height as the shoulders.

Repeat three to twelve times.

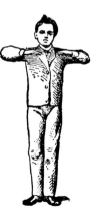

(FIG. 58) STANDING, SWIMMING

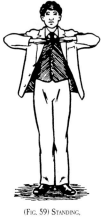

(FIG. 59) STANDING,
ARMS-FLINGING, BACKWARD I

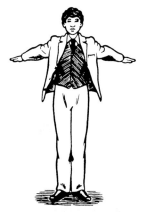

(FIG. 60) STANDING,
ARMS-FLINGING, BACKWARD II

Exercise 34: Standing, Arms-Flinging, Backward

Take the same initial position *(Fig. 59)* as described for swimming (Exercise 33). With one movement quickly throw the arms backward as far as possible, still keeping them at the same height as the shoulders *(Fig. 60)*.

This is an excellent exercise to develop the chest and increase the breathing capacity.

Repeat three to twelve times.

Exercise 35: Standing, Fingers-Bending & Extending.

Clench both hands and then extend the fingers alternately *(Figs. 61 to 63)*. Considerable vigour should be put into these flexions and extensions.

Repeat three to twelve times.

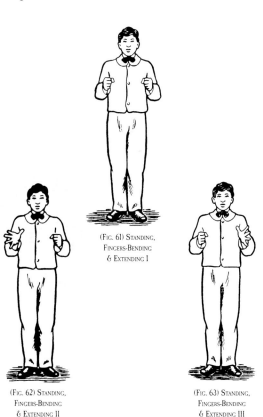

(Fig. 61) Standing,
Fingers-Bending
& Extending I

(Fig. 62) Standing,
Fingers-Bending
& Extending II

(Fig. 63) Standing,
Fingers-Bending
& Extending III

" The man who is blessed with firm, elastic muscles and an erect carriage possesses a formidable equipment for the battle of life "

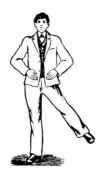

Chapter 6

Leg & Foot Movements

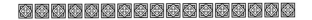

SIMPLE LEG & FOOT MOVEMENTS

Leg and Foot Movements.

Many of these movements require careful balancing and hence must be taken very accurately. There is always a tendency to neglect the position of the trunk in doing leg movements, but this is a mistake. The trunk should be kept erect, as described in the correct standing position *(Fig. 64)*.

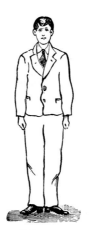

(FIG. 64) CORRECT STANDING

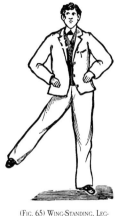

(Fig. 65) Wing-Standing, Leg-Extending, Sideward I

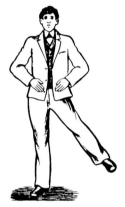

(Fig. 66) Wing-Standing, Leg-Extending, Sideward II

Exercise 36: Wing-Standing, Leg-Extending, Sideward.

Extend the right leg to the same side as far and as high as possible. In taking this and similar movements, do not allow the body to sway to the opposite side, but constantly maintain the erect position of the trunk *(Fig. 65)*.

Do the same with the left leg *(Fig. 66)*.

Then alternate right and left.

Repeat each movement two to six times.

Exercise 37: Standing, Leg-Extending.

Forward.

Extend the right leg straight forward as high as possible, keeping the knee extended, and maintaining the correct poise of trunk.

Extend the left leg in the same way; then alternately right and left, repeating each movement two to six times *(Figs. 67 to 68)*.

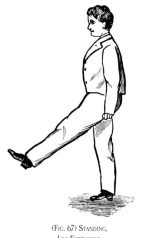

(Fig. 67) Standing,
Leg-Extending,
Forward (Left Leg)

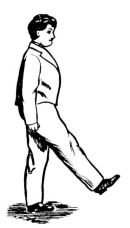

(Fig. 68) Standing,
Leg-Extending,
Forward (Right Leg)

Backward.

Extend the right leg backward as far as possible, again keeping both knees straight, and the trunk erect *(Figs. 69 and 70).* Do likewise with the left leg *(Figs. 71 and 72),* and then alternately, right and left.

Repeat two to six times.

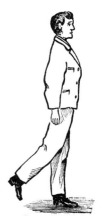

(Fig. 69) Standing, Leg-Extending, Backward (Right Leg)

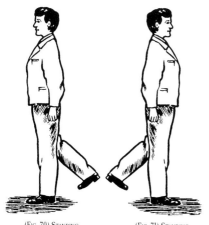

(Fig. 70) Standing, Leg-Extending, Backward (Right Leg)

(Fig. 71) Standing, Leg-Extending, Backward (Left Leg)

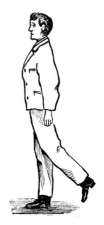

(Fig. 72) Standing, Leg-Extending, Backward (Left Leg)

Exercise 38: Wing-Standing, Leg-Twisting.

While standing on the right leg, raise the left slightly and twist it vigorously to the left, keeping the knee extended; then to the right, and alternately, repeating each movement two to six times *(Figs. 73 to 75)*. Do likewise with the right leg *(Figs. 76 to 78)*.

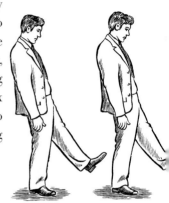

(FIG. 73) WING-STANDING, LEG-TWISTING I

(FIG. 74) WING-STANDING LEG-TWISTING II

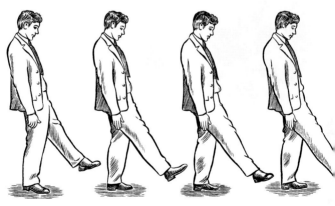

(FIG. 75) WING-STANDING, LEG-TWISTING III

(FIG. 76) WING-STANDING, LEG-TWISTING IV

(FIG. 77) WING-STANDING, LEG-TWISTING V

(FIG. 78) WING-STAND LEG-TWISTING VI

Exercise 39: Standing, Leg-Lifting & Standing, Leg-Bending.

Leg-Lifting.

Raise the right leg forward, so that there will be a right angle at the hip-joint, and also at the knee-joint *(Fig. 79)*. Now raise the left leg in the same way *(Fig. 80)*.

Repeat each three to twelve times.

Leg-Bending.

Bend the right leg so that a right angle is formed at the knee. The thigh is to be kept parallel with the other limb *(Fig. 81)*.

Bend the left leg in the same way *(Fig. 82)*.

Repeat each three to twelve times.

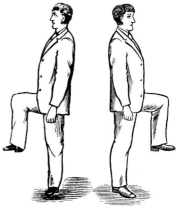

(FIG. 79)
STANDING, LEG-LIFTING I

(FIG. 80)
STANDING, LEG-LIFTING II

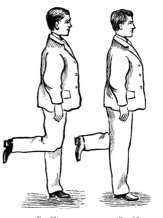

(FIG. 81)
STANDING, LEG-BENDING I

(FIG. 82)
STANDING, LEG-BENDING II

Exercise 40: Wing-Standing, Knee-Bending
& Wing-Standing, Heel-Raising.

Knee-Bending.

Bend the knees to a right angle, if possible, keeping
the heels firmly on the ground, and the trunk erect
(Figs. 83 to 85).

Repeat three to twelve times.

Heel-Raising.

Rise on the toes as high as possible *(Figs. 86 to 87)*.

Repeat three to twelve times.

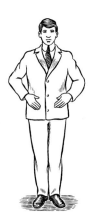

(Fig. 83)
Wing-Standing,
Knee-Bending I

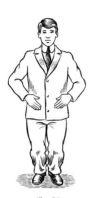

(Fig. 84)
WING-STANDING,
KNEE-BENDING II

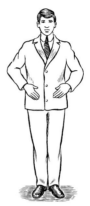

(Fig. 85)
WING-STANDING,
KNEE-BENDING III

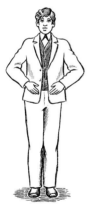

(Fig. 86)
WING-STANDING,
HEEL-RAISING I

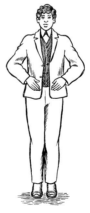

(Fig. 87)
WING-STANDING,
HEEL-RAISING II

✻✻✻✻✻

" The training of the muscles, kept within the proper limits, enlivens the spirits and the general tone of a person, mentally as well as physically "

✻✻✻✻✻

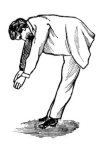

Chapter 7

Combined
Exercise

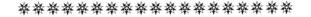

COMBINATION OF
MOVEMENTS

The foregoing exercises may be combined with different positions, which give variety and render the exercises more or less difficult. For example, head-bending may be taken in the ordinary standing position (Exercise 1) or in certain compound positions, such as: close-standing, a little more vigorous; toe-standing, requiring still more energy; wing-standing, a comfortable and easy position; bend-standing; heave-standing, a little more difficult; rest-standing, more difficult; and stretch-standing, more vigorous. These various positions are fully described in Exercises 2 to 10 inclusive. Some of them may also be combined with the sitting and lying primary positions, thus giving a still larger variety of exercises, and allowing them to be graded according to the physical condition of the individual case.

Several exercises, too, may be combined together. For example, arm-raising with heel-raising. Space forbids us to give more than a very few of these compound exercises, but the number may be augmented almost indefinitely.

DAILY PROGRAMME

The following programme of exercises has been prepared for those who wish to do them systematically. There are ten groups, and each group may be taken daily or twice daily for a week or longer.

Day	Exercise Number											
1	19	20	11	25	40	12	27	39	28	11		
11	19	21	25	13	28	36	29	40	35	11	33	
111	19	22	26	14	32	37	30	13	38	34	39	11
1V	19	22	23	31	12	32	37	33	11	39	26	
V	19	20	21	28	13	29	40	32	12	28	40	
V1	19	20	22	25	12	37	34	16	39	14	27	
V11	19	24	21	28	13	33	38	43	42	11		
V111	24	20	11	28	14	36	35	32	46	49		
1X	24	21	23	42	47	41	14	45	44	48	34	40
X	24	21	43	50	39	33	13	35	40	32	47	

RISING ON TOES

Exercise 41: Standing, Arms-Stretching with Heel-Raising.

This is the same as Exercise 27, except that each time both arms are stretched the gymnast rises on his toes *(Figs. 88 to 91)*. Repeat two to six times.

Exercise 42: Close-Standing, Arms-Raising.

See Exercise 2 for the initial position. Raise the arms as directed in Exercises 25, and 26.

Exercise 43: Wing-Close-Standing, Heel-Raising.

The initial position is a combination of wing-standing and close-standing (see Exercises 2 and 5). Raise the heels as high as possible from the floor.

Repeat three to twelve times.

Exercise 44: Bend-Close-Standing, Arm-Extending.

This is a combination of bend-standing (Exercise 6) and close-standing (Exercise 2). For further directions for the procedure, see Exercise 28.

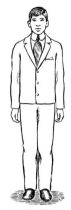

(Fig. 88)
STANDING, ARMS-STRETCHING
WITH HEEL-RAISING I

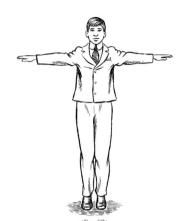

(Fig. 89)
STANDING, ARMS-STRETCHING
WITH HEEL-RAISING II

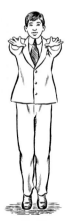

(Fig. 90)
STANDING, ARMS-STRETCHING
WITH HEEL-RAISING III

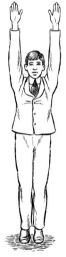

(Fig. 91)
STANDING, ARMS-STRETCHING
WITH HEEL-RAISING IV

HANDS ON HIPS

Exercise 45: Wing-Toe-Close-Standing, Knee-Bending.

The initial position is a combination of toe and close-standing with the hands on the hips (wing-position).

For the movement see Exercise 40.

Exercise 46: Rest-Close-Standing, Heel-Raising.

The initial position is a combination of rest and close-standing (Exercises 2 and 8).

Many other movements may be taken from this position, such as Exercises 12, 13, 14 and 39.

Exercise 47: Rest-Toe-Standing, Trunk-Bending.

Here we have a combination of rest and toe-standing (Exercises 3 and 8).

For the trunk-bendings see Exercises 12 to 13.

Other movements may also be taken from this position, such as Exercises 36 to 40.

Exercise 48: Wing-Sitting, Head-Bending/
Wing-Sitting, Knees-Opening & Closing.

Head-Bending.

The hands are placed upon the hips the same as in wing-standing.

For the exercise see Exercise 11.

Knees-Opening & Closing.

Separate the knees a foot or more, and close them again. The heels should remain touching during the exercise *(Figs. 92 and 93)*.

Repeat three to twelve times.

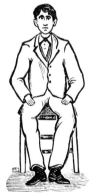

(FIG. 92) WING-SITTING,
KNEES-OPENING & CLOSING I

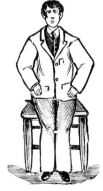

(FIG. 93) WING-SITTING,
KNEES-OPENING & CLOSING II

VIGOROUS EXERCISES

Exercise 49:
Wing-Toe-Standing, Jumping.

This and the following exercises are quite vigorous and proper care should be taken to avoid strain or over-exertion.

The initial position is a combination of wing-standing and toe-standing. Bend the knees to a right angle, and then make a light jump in place, coming down on your toes, and with knees bent *(Figs. 94 to 97)*.

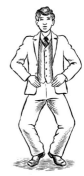

(Fig. 94)
WING-TOE-STANDING,
JUMPING I

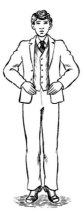

(Fig. 95)
WING-TOE-STANDING,
JUMPING II

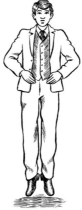

(Fig. 96)
WING-TOE-STANDING,
JUMPING III

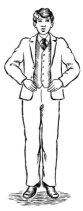

(Fig. 97)
WING-TOE-STANDING,
JUMPING IV

Repeat two to six times.

This exercise may be varied by jumping forward, sideward, or backward *(Figs. 98 to 101)*.

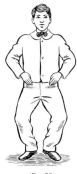

(Fig. 98)
WING-TOE-STANDING,
JUMPING, SIDEWARD I

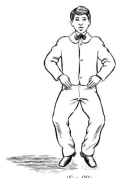

(Fig. 99)
WING-TOE-STANDING,
JUMPING, SIDEWARD II

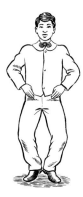

(Fig. 100)
WING-TOE-STANDING,
JUMPING, BACKWARD

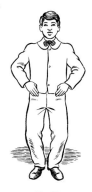

(Fig. 101)
WING-TOE-STANDING,
JUMPING, FORWARD

BENDING & FLEXING

The development of a supple and strong physique brings with it the resultant benefits of improved posture and greater overall physical well-being.

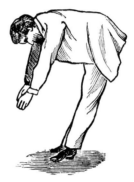

(Fig. 102) Stretch-Standing, Trunk-Bending, Forward

Exercise 50: Stretch-Standing, Trunk-Bending, Forward.

Take the correct position and bend forward and downward, trying to touch the floor with the fingers. If impossible to touch the floor at first, practice will soon make it easy *(Fig. 102)*. Avoid straining.

Repeat two to six times.

Flexion and Resistance.

In concluding the exercises, we will briefly describe a very simple yet effective method, which we may call flexion or extension with resistance.

Bend the fingers of the right hand slowly, at the same time opposing the flexion by the extensor muscles. It is possible to put considerable energy into the exercise. After complete flexion, extend the fingers slowly, at the same time opposing extension by the flexor muscles *(Fig. 103)*.

If both hands are closed at the same time, and then the wrists and elbows flexed in turn, the movement becomes a very powerful one. Any group of flexor or extensor muscles may be exercised in the same way.

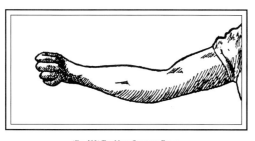

(Fig. 103) The Hand Strongly Flexed

❋❋❋❋

" Take the daily cold bath. In winter it will probably be best to take it as a wet-hand rub, or sponge bath, always followed by vigorous friction "

❋❋❋❋

Chapter 8
Personal Hygiene & Well-being

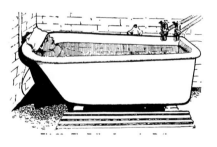

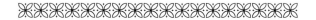

Teeth, Nails & Skin

"Nature's Food Filter," or The New System of
Thorough Mastication, or "Fletcherising."

For many years, "masticate thoroughly" has been a common expression with physicians; but usually it has not meant much. Mr. Horace Fletcher, however, has reduced chewing to a fine art, and his system has benefited so many, and appeals so strongly to one's common sense, that it calls for some consideration in a work on health culture.

Mr. Fletcher began his experiments in 1898, when he was afflicted with "over-robustness" and suffered from allied disorders of a sufficiently grave character to render him ineligible for life insurance. What led him to give special attention to mastication we do not know; but his system consists in what he dubs "Nature's Food Filter," a method, called "Fletcherising," that does not allow the swallowing of food of any sort until thorough mastication has deprived it of all its flavours, and reduced it to a fine liquid. Any stringy, indigestible matter which may still remain in the mouth is then rejected. Water only is to be drunk, being tasteless.

After following this plan for only three months, Mr. Fletcher found that his appetite was fully appeased with less than half the amount of food he had been in the habit of taking. Moreover, his weight decreased from 205 lbs. to 163 lbs., while his strength increased. Mr. Fletcher, it may be said in passing, is in sympathy with vegetarian principles. "Much meat," he says in a recent publication, "excites lust, intemperance, and savagery in man."

If it be thought that living on half the ordinary rations must cause weakness, it may be answered that Mr. Fletcher on his 50th birthday took a bicycle ride of 304 kilometres.

Time Required for Meals.

Mr. Fletcher eats but two meals daily, and finds forty-five minutes' chewing sufficient, so the amount of time required is not nearly so great as one would think.

If men are eating double the amount of food needed, it is reasonable to believe that a great deal of energy, which might be utilised in useful mental or physical labour, is expended in ridding the system of the surplus nutrition.

In conclusion, we heartily commend the idea to our readers, especially those who are suffering from digestive disorders.

The Nails.

Unclean finger-nails are not only distinctly disagreeable to the eye, and suggestive of bad breeding, but they are full of danger to the individual himself and to others. Numerous colonies of disease germs nestle in the filth to be found under neglected finger-nails, and cases of serious infection have been thus caused, though in the vast majority of cases the evil done in this way might very likely be charged to other causes. Warm water and soap, with the industrious use of the nail brush and attention to proper trimming, will usually ensure a clean and healthy condition of the nails of both hands and feet. The former, it may be said in passing, should be cut round, the latter should be cut across to avoid painful ingrowing.

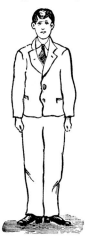

(Fig. 104) It is Not Well to Over-Clothe the Body

The Clothing.

A great deal has been said in favour of woollen underclothing, but for persons in reasonably vigorous health it is coming to be considered that linen mesh garments afford the ideal material to put next to the skin. Such fabrics, while they do not have the cold clammy "feel" of closely-woven linen, receive and throw off quickly all moisture from the body, thus keeping the skin dry and clean, whereas the woollen underwear, by retaining the moisture, encourages a relaxed state of the skin, which destroys its natural resistive powers against change of temperature.

Evils of Over-Clothing.

It is not well to over-clothe the body *(Fig. 104)*. Heavy coverlets by night, and too much clothing by day are likely to interfere decidedly with an alert, vigorous condition of the body. It does not make for comfort in the long run, for the more the body is coddled, the more sensitive does it become to the cold. Sometimes a process of hardening is an excellent thing. One excellent means of improving the tone of the skin is the air bath. Disrobe completely, and give the whole body a vigorous rubbing with a flesh brush or with the bare hand. Light gymnastics may also be taken during the air bath.

Baths.

Habits of strict personal cleanliness are of the greatest importance in the maintenance of health. Not less than one warm bath weekly, with plenty of soap and vigorous application of the flesh brush, are required for this purpose. The daily cold bath also helps to keep the skin in a clean, wholesome condition; and should be taken in some form by everyone who would keep himself "fit". A cold bath should never be taken immediately after eating, neither is a very warm bath desirable at such a time. Most people find the early morning hour the best time for the cold bath or douche or the wet-towel rub. The warm or hot bath is taken to advantage in the evening just before the moment of retiring.

Malodorous Sweat.

Some persons very cleanly in their habits are troubled with malodorous perspiration. Sometimes the cause is to be found in an inactive condition of the bowels or other eliminating organs, by which an extra burden is thrown on the skin. Of course, such conditions must first be removed. Frequent warm baths with plenty of good soap, and the morning cold bath, together with wholesome habits in general, will then usually bring about a cure. Dusting the armpits with a mixture of borax and talcum powder will be found helpful.

Frequent change of underwear is also essential, and care should be taken to clothe the body lightly, giving free access to the air. Too much clothing is extremely favourable to abnormal activity of the sweat glands.

Hydrotherapy in the Home.

The treatment of disease by the use of water in one form or another is not a modern discovery. The Japanese, Chinese, and other ancient nations have utilised water in this way for many centuries. The famous Grecian physician, Hippocrates, who lived nearly two thousand years ago, recommended baths in the treatment of physical ailments. However, for hundreds of years during the Dark Ages but little attention was paid to the use of water, and hydrotherapy almost became a lost art. Priessnitz, of Germany, may be regarded as the father of modern hydrotherapy. He was a simple peasant, who, like Sir Isaac Newton, had learned the value of observation. His early experience with water as a remedial agency reads almost like a romance. Later, Dr. Winternitz, of Vienna, and others, took up the supposedly new treatment and developed it. Dr. Kellogg, of the Battle Creek Sanitarium, was among the first to reduce water treatment to a science. He made a large number of careful scientific experiments, the results of which are given in his admirable book, "Rational Hydrotherapy."

" A tepid or cool sponge bath, followed by vigorous friction, should be administered at once, after which the patient should go to bed "

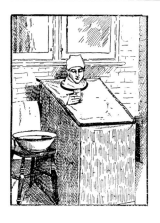

Chapter 9

Baths & Bathing

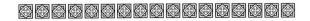

TYPES OF BATH

The Full or Immersion Bath.

This is one of the most comfortable of baths as far as position is concerned. The person lies on his back in an easy position, and relaxes his limbs and muscles. This relaxation is essential to the most favourable results. The water should cover the chest, and reach to the chin. In giving a hot bath it is well to apply a cold compress to the head. A towel wrung out of cold water may be arranged in the form of a turban. The duration of the bath varies according to the temperature. Five minutes is usually long enough for a hot bath. A warm bath may occupy a period of ten or fifteen minutes.

On leaving a warm or hot bath of any description, a cold application of some kind is advisable. A cold spray, if available, gives an excellent finishing touch; but simpler means may be used; such as a tepid or cold sponge, a wet hand rub, or a cold mitten friction. These procedures are more fully described in the proceeding chapters.

The Neutral Full Bath (92° to 97° Fahr.).

The temperature of the water should be about 97° or 98° Fahr. to begin with, and afterward gradually lowered several degrees. As the term "neutral" indicates, the water should be neither hot nor cold. The bath is pleasant, producing a feeling of comfort and well-being *(Fig. 105)*.

The ordinary neutral bath lasts from ten to thirty minutes, but it may be prolonged almost indefinitely when required, thus making it useful in treating severe and extensive burns of the skin. It is an excellent means of relieving insomnia—the patient should be sent directly to bed if used for this purpose—and is effectual in treating hysteria, neurasthenia, anaemia, chlorosis, mild forms of insanity, and various other ills.

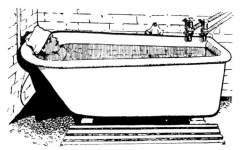

(Fig. 105) The Neutral Full Bath

Shallow Bath with Attendant.

The temperature of the water is warm, neutral, or tepid, and the quantity is merely sufficient to cover the thighs. The attendant applies vigorous friction to the back while pouring on the cold water *(Fig. 106)*.

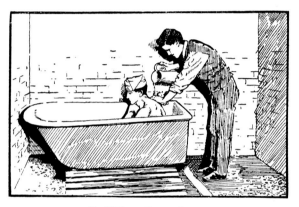

(Fig. 106) Shallow Bath with Attendant

The Sitz or Hip Baths.

For these baths a sitz tub is required. The bath may be hot, warm, neutral, or any temperature desired. The hot sitz bath is often indicated for inflammatory disorders of the pelvic organs.

A hot foot bath is usually given in combination with sitz baths *(Fig. 107)*.

The neutral sitz bath is similar in its effects to the neutral full bath, but milder.

The rubbing sitz is a tepid or cool bath which is given with vigorous friction to the immersed parts of the body. It may occupy from one to five minutes, according to the temperature of the water. It is recommended for piles and constipation.

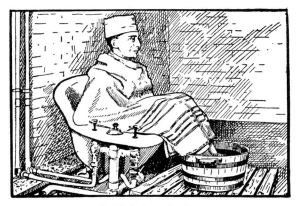

(FIG. 107) THE SITZ AND FOOT BATH

The Hot Foot Bath
(105° to 120° Fahr., 5 to 20 minutes).

A very simple bath, easy to administer, and efficacious in its results, is the hot foot bath. It may be given in any room of the house. Provide plenty of boiling water. Give the bath as hot as the patient will stand, and add more hot water every few minutes. The patient may drink two or three glasses of hot water or hot lemonade to advantage during the bath *(Fig. 108)*.

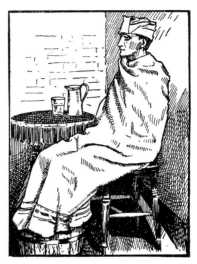

(FIG. 108) THE HOT FOOT BATH

Bathe the face and head with cold water, and apply a cold compress to the head. Have a temperature of 105°Fahr. to begin with, and gradually increase to 115°or 120°. If necessary, wrap the patient in a blanket to keep him warm. The bath should continue until there is free perspiration. On taking the feet out of the bath, pour cold water over them and dry well.

Uses of the Hot Foot Bath.

The hot foot bath is an excellent remedy for a cold in the head, a sore throat, or a mild case of influenza; a sprain or dislocation of the ankle; also for neuralgia, rheumatism and gout of the feet. By drawing the blood into the lower limbs it acts as a derivative and often relieves a congestive headache. It always helps to equalise the circulation; consequently it is a remedy for cold feet.

By drawing blood from the head, it renders the brain anaemic and so favours sleep. Indeed, it affords great relief in certain forms of insomnia. The hot foot bath is also highly recommended for the treatment of dyspepsia and indigestion.

To intensify this bath, two tablespoonfuls of ground mustard may be added to the water. This is called a mustard foot bath.

Water Temperatures	
degrees Fahrenheit	
less than 32	Freezing
32–50	Very cold
50–70	Cold
70–80	Cold
80–92	Tepid
92–97	Neutral
97–102	Warm
102–105	Hot
more than 105	Very hot

The Hot Leg Bath. (105° to 120° Fahr.).

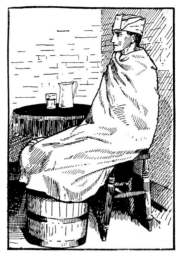

(FIG. 109) THE HOT LEG BATH

For this a deeper tub is required, as the water should reach nearly up to the knees; otherwise the procedure is quite the same as for a foot bath, and the uses are very much the same *(Fig. 109)*.

The Alternate Hot and Cold Foot Bath
(110° to 120° and 40° to 50° Fahr.).

For this bath two foot tubs will be required, one containing hot and the other cold water. After soaking the feet in hot water for two to three minutes, transfer them to the cold water for twenty or thirty seconds, and then back to the hot water. This process may be repeated four to six times, after which the feet are dried from the cold bath. Keep up the temperature of the hot water by the addition of boiling water from time to time.

This bath has a more powerful effect upon the circulation than the plain foot bath, and is one of the best preventative measures against cold feet, sweating feet, and chilblains.

An alternate hot and cold leg bath may be given in like manner, except that two leg tubs are used instead of foot tubs *(Fig. 110)*.

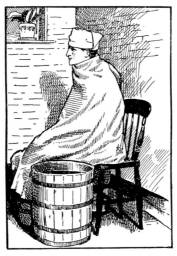

(Fig. 110) The Alternate Hot and Cold Leg Bath

The Arm Bath
(105° to 120° Fahr.).

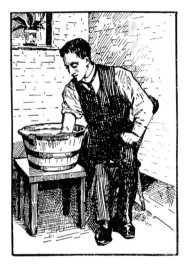

(Fig. III) Arm Bath

This is a simple form of bath, and not difficult to give. It is rarely resorted to except for a sprain of the wrist, chronic ulceration of the arm, or extensive burning. The bath may be given in a large basin or other suitable vessel *(Fig. 111)*. If a continuous bath, the arm should be occasionally dipped in cold water for an instant; then returned to the hot bath.

Elbow or hand baths may also be administered for special reasons.

The Hot Air Bath
(5 to 20 minutes, 120° to 200° Fahr.).

A specially prepared cabinet is useful for the hot air bath, but not essential. The treatment may be given by placing the patient on a cane-seated chair, under which a burning lamp is placed. A piece of metal must be fitted under the seat to prevent burning. The patient is then well wrapped in sheet and blankets, which retain the hot air. But this method is not to be generally recommended, for, even with the best of care, there is always danger of setting the clothing or chair on fire.

A good cabinet bath is far better, and can be obtained for a reasonable sum. The air is heated by an alcohol lamp, petroleum, or gas, and care must be taken to prevent burning, because, even with the best constructed cabinets, there is still some danger of fire if proper precautions are not observed. Have the bath cabinet warm before introducing the patient. Give a pint or more of hot water to drink during the bath. This facilitates perspiration, and renders the treatment more effective. Bathe the face and head in cold water, and apply a cold compress to the head. This should be changed every five minutes.

The feet may be placed in hot water or on a hot brick during the bath.

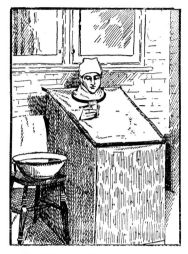

(FIG. 112) CABINET FOR HOT AIR OR VAPOUR BATHS

The hot air bath is followed by a cold sponge, cold mitten friction, or cold full bath and friction.

This is an efficient remedy for a cold, influenza, bronchitis, rheumatic disorders, especially lumbago, sciatica, acute and chronic Bright's disease (except where the patient has reached the advanced stage), and obesity.

The hot air bath is to be avoided in fevers, and where there is extreme weakness of the heart.

The Hot Vapour Bath
(5 to 20 minutes, 110° to 120° Fahr.).

This is similar to the foregoing except that, instead of dry, hot air, there is hot vapour or wet steam. Like the hot air bath, it is also given in a specially prepared cabinet. By means of a suitable lamp, water is boiled, and the steam produced furnishes the hot vapour. Again careful precautions must be taken to avoid the incidence of fire (*Fig. 112*).

The patient is encouraged to drink a pint of hot water. A cold application, such as the cold mitten friction, the cold spray, or shower, follows the bath, after which the patient is dried, and an oil rub administered if desired.

The hot vapour bath is useful for the various disorders mentioned under the hot air bath, and also for neurasthenia, neuralgia, hypochondria, hysteria, and obesity. But it must be avoided in cases of severe heart or kidney disease.

The Electric Light Bath (5 to 20 minutes).

This paragon of hot baths is the invention of Dr. J.H. Kellogg. It is the cleanest, pleasantest, and most convenient known, and in time will probably displace both Turkish and Russian baths. It can be administered either sitting or recumbent, with the head included or excluded; or it may be administered locally to the spine, abdomen, or one of the limbs (*Fig. 113*).

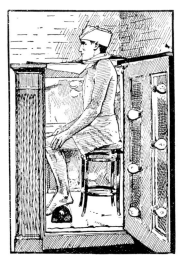

(Fig. 113) Electric Light Bath Cabinet

There are various forms of the electric light or radiant heat bath, the most common form being a cabinet fitted with ordinary incandescent burners. But the arc light may also be used, as well as red or blue lights, for special purposes.

A cold compress is folded about the head to prevent faintness, and the patient remains in the bath five to eight minutes for tonic effects, and longer for eliminative purposes. On leaving the bath, some form of cold application is always given to the patient to close the pores of the skin and prevent taking cold. An oil rub is a good finishing procedure.

EFFECTS OF RADIANT HEAT

The radiant energy of the electric light has a remarkably penetrating power, and reaches the tissues beneath the skin with great ease. In this respect it is vastly superior to the hot air or vapour bath.

A brief electric light bath is useful for its tonic effects. These, although mild, are nevertheless very real and effective, the patient feeling exhilarated and strengthened by them.

When the bath is sufficiently prolonged, the eliminative effects are powerful; heat applied in this form being one of the best reducing agents available. Consequently the treatment is suitable for persons suffering with diabetes, obesity, syphilis, neuralgia, eczema, migraine, neurasthenia, hysteria, and all rheumatic and gouty disorders. It is also useful in anaemia, and in various forms of indigestion, especially nervous dyspepsia.

The radiant heat bath may be recommended for people engaged in sedentary occupations, for whom it is an efficient preventative of many ailments.

❋❋❋❋❋

" Inflammations of all kinds can usually be treated
to advantage by fomentations, and these hot cloths
can easily be applied to any part of the body "

❋❋❋❋❋

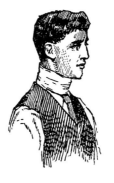

Chapter 10

Compresses & Fomentations

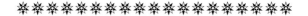

TYPES OF COMPRESS

The Compress.

There are many forms of the compress that are used in treating disease, but we shall confine our attention to the most common and useful varieties only. The compress may be defined as an application of water by means of a cloth. Wool, linen, and cotton, especially the first two, are most commonly used. The poultice is really an old-fashioned form of compress, but is less clean and less convenient. It will ultimately fall out of use.

Two to four or six thicknesses of linen, or double the number of layers of butter muslin may be used. For hot applications flannel is usually preferred.

A compress may be hot or cold, or any intermediate temperature. The degree of heat largely determines the effect upon the body.

The Fomentation.

As the term itself indicates, this is a hot compress. It is one of the most useful of water treatments, and is both inexpensive and easily prepared. According to Dr. Kellogg, "it is essentially a local vapour bath."

Fomentation cloths are readily prepared by dividing an ordinary large woollen blanket into four equal parts. If the same part of the body is to be repeatedly treated, it is well to oil the skin with coconut butter as a protection.

The patient usually lies on a couch while undergoing treatment, and is covered with a sheet and a blanket. Have a pail of boiling water ready. Fold the fomentation cloth so that there will four thicknesses over the part to be treated; again fold once or twice lengthwise; grasp one end of the cloth in each hand, give it a turn or two, and dip in the hot water; then wring out by twisting and pulling the ends apart. The fomentation cloth must be wrung out thoroughly and smartly to save dripping and loss of heat.

Fomenting the Hips.

Suppose the hips are to be treated. Have the patient lie on his face, and place a single layer of dry flannel over the hips. Then lay the fomentation cloth over this. Press it down snugly against the body, and cover with a dry flannel after folding back the ends, to retain the heat. The fomentation is left in place for five minutes and then replaced by another, which is retained for five minutes, to give place to a third and final. Each succeeding application is hotter than the previous. They should be as hot as can be borne, but sufficient care should be taken to avoid blistering the skin *(Fig. 114)*.

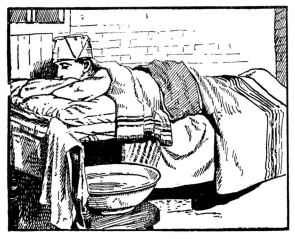

(Fig. 114) Fomentation to the Hips

On removing the last fomentation, the surface treated should present a scarlet red colour. Bathe the part with cold water and dry gently. The treatment can be repeated in an hour or after a longer period, according to the circumstances of the case.

Inflammations of all kinds can usually be treated to advantage by fomentations, and these hot cloths can easily be applied to any part of the body. They are most useful in treating acute and chronic stomach disorders, torpid livers, sprains, bruises, dislocations, fractures, renal and hepatic colic, neuralgia, constipation, rheumatic and gouty joints, lumbago and many other ailments.

Hot Foot Baths and
Fomentations to the Spine.

Oftentimes various separate procedures, such as fomentations to the spine or some other part of the body, are combined with the hot foot bath for the purpose of producing more marked results. The water must be as hot as can be borne, and a cold compress is applied to the head as a matter of course. The duration of the combined treatments is from ten to twenty minutes, being governed largely by the circumstances of the case *(Fig. 115)*.

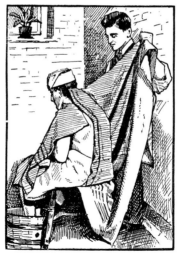

(Fig. 115) Hot Foot Bath

The Mustard Fomentation.

To intensify the effect and increase counter-irritation ground mustard may be added in the proportion of a tablespoonful to a quart of water. The mustard is steeped in the water, which is then poured over the fomentation cloth, the latter being wrung out as usual and applied to the body. Take care to avoid blistering, especially where the skin is tender and sensitive. The mustard fomentation is very effective in relieving severe pain.

The Rubber Bottle Fomentation.

Continuous moist heat can easily be provided by placing a rubber water bottle, half full of very hot water, over the fomentation. This saves changing the fomentation every five minutes, and is quite as successful in many cases. Every hour, or oftener, the fomentation should be removed and a cold compress applied for a few minutes, after which the fomentation may be resumed.

The Hot Water Rubber Bottle.

This is a most convenient means of applying dry heat to the body. The bottle should not be more than one-half full, otherwise it will be very difficult to adjust it snugly to the skin. Press out the air before closing the mouth. The hot water bottle is a simple and effective means of relieving inflammatory affections, bruises, sprains, neuralgia, rheumatism and similar affections.

The Heating Compress.

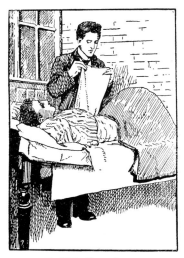

(Fig. 116) The Heating Compress
Applying the Moist Towel

This consists of a linen compress covered with two or three layers of flannel, which overlap above and below, and therefore hinder the entrance of air and prevent chilling. A linen towel of suitable size serves the purpose very well. Wring it rather dry out of cold water, and apply snugly to the body, say around the chest or abdomen. Then wrap with the dry flannel. It is usually left in place for several hours or overnight. On removing, bathe the part with cold water and dry well *(Figs. 116 to 117)*.

The physiological effect is to cause a large flow of blood to the affected part. The cold sensation passes away quickly, and is followed by a feeling of warmth and comfort.

The heating compress is successful in relieving chronic catarrh of the throat, chronic bronchitis, and various gastric and intestinal disturbances. Applied to the stomach and bowels, it is called the abdominal girdle, and becomes a most powerful remedy for chronic dyspepsia, intestinal catarrh, constipation, sluggish liver, chronic backache, and prolapse and dilatation of the stomach.

If used daily, the compress should be boiled between each treatment to keep it clean. Otherwise it may give rise to an eruption of the skin.

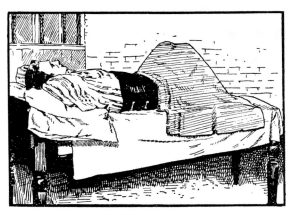

(Fig. 117) Heating Compress
Moist Towel Fastened in Position and Flannel Band Adjusted

The Cooling Compress.

The compress should be maintained at a constant temperature of 55°to 70°Fahr. This can be achieved by frequent changing. The effect is distinctly sedative. It is useful in typhoid fever, and also in certain forms of inflammation.

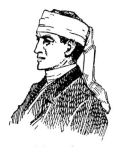

(Fig. 118) Cooling Compress
Application to the Head

The Cold Compress.

In giving almost any hot bath or hot treatment, it is customary to apply a cold compress to the head. The procedure is as follows. First, bathe the head and face and also the neck, if desired, with cold water. Next, wring a towel or a piece of linen of suitable size out of cold water, so that it still remains fairly wet, and apply it to the head in the form of a turban. This should be changed for a fresh one as frequently as it becomes warm; ordinarily, at least every five minutes. It should not be so wet as to permit of water trickling down over the face or neck, which is very unpleasant *(Fig. 118)*.

The cold compress has a pleasant, soothing effect upon the patient. It prevents faintness, and helps to equalise the circulation of the blood.

The cold compress is also helpful in stopping nose bleeding and other haemorrhages, and relives neuralgia better than heat in some cases. It should not be applied continuously for more than half or three-quarters of an hour. Then it should be interrupted by a fomentation for five minutes, which will bring back the natural heat, and prevent untoward results.

Cold Compress to the Neck.

Take a small linen towel of suitable size, and fold it lengthwise, so that the folds are about two or three inches wide. Soak it in cold or ice water, and wring well. Apply it snugly to the neck, and fasten by safety pins *(Fig. 119)*. Next cover the moist towel by two or three thicknesses of flannel, so that the dry flannel overlaps above and below, preventing the access of air. The flannel needs to be applied snugly and fastened with pins *(Fig. 120)*. On removing the compress, bathe the neck with cold water and dry well.

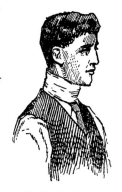

(Fig. 119) Cold Compress
Application to the Neck.
The Moist Towels

It is a good plan to apply the cold compress at night, and remove it in the morning. This makes an excellent treatment for chronic sore throat.

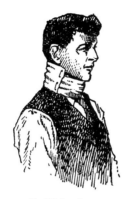

(Fig. 120) Cold Compress
Application to the Neck. The Dry Flannel Covering

"Hot and Cold" to the Spine.

First apply a fomentation for five minutes, and then a cold compress for thirty to sixty seconds. Repeat three to six times. Finish with the cold compress.

This treatment is very useful for neurasthenia, hysteria, insomnia, and other nervous disorders.

The usefulness of the alternate hot and cold compress is not confined to the spine; it may also be applied to other parts of the body. For bedsores, paralysed limbs, alcoholic intoxication, and for local exciting and stimulating effects generally, it is a valuable form of treatment.

❝ Sleep on a hard bed. Follow a wholesome diet, eating largely dry, hard foods. Avoid cheap novels and exciting stories ❞

.

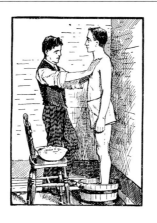

Chapter 11

Tonic Measures

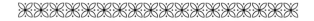

SPONGE & RUB

Tepid or Cold Wet Hand Rub.

This makes one of the mildest of tonic remedies if tepid water is used. The water should be from 40° to 80° Fahr. Even iced water may be used. Have several Turkish towels to hand. Place the patient on a couch, wrapped in a sheet and blanket. Expose each part of the body as required. Begin with the chest,

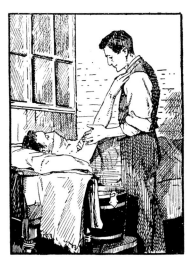

(FIG. 121) WET HAND RUB

116

which is quickly bathed with the hands, care being used not to spatter water in the patient's face. Then dry quickly, leaving a red glow of warmth. Cover the chest and proceed to the abdomen, right and left arms, right and left legs, and finally the back. The treatment must be given briskly to accomplish the most good, and each part should only occupy a few seconds *(Fig. 121)*.

The tepid or cold wet hand rub is a first class method of reducing temperature and increasing vital resistance. It is especially adapted to children and the aged because of its exceedingly mild nature.

The Cold Sponge (50° to 70° Fahr.).

Have the patient standing in hot water (105° Fahr.) and, by means of a sponge or small Turkish towel, go over the body rapidly, then wrap in a dry sheet, and rub vigorously. Bathe the face with cold water on leaving the foot tub. The cold sponge may be taken by the patient without assistance, or given by an attendant *(Fig. 122)*.

Although a mild tonic, it is a much more vigorous treatment than the wet hand rub. It is a valuable measure in anaemia, chlorosis, nervous debility, general malnutrition, and dropsy.

A cool or cold sponge is a most effective means of treating fevers, especially in children, the aged, and the feeble patients.

The Tepid Sponge (80° to 90° Fahr.).

This is a still milder tonic, and very useful for relieving light fevers. Given gently, it is an excellent means of refreshing anyone who is tired or worn out *(Fig. 122)*.

The Hot Sponge (120° to 140° Fahr.).

The sponge should not be moist enough to drop water, and the treatment should be administered quickly. The patient may be lying on a couch or standing, as desired. It is recommended for relieving night sweats. If vinegar or alcohol in equal parts be added, the results are still more satisfactory.

The Cold Mitten Friction (32° to 50° Fahr.).

Cold or ice-cold water may be used, according to the case and the effects desired.

A well-fitting mitten made of Russell cord, coarse mohair, or some other rough cloth, is wetted in cold water and rubbed briskly over the skin. Vigorous friction is desirable in order to produce the best results. The patient lies down on a couch and is covered with a sheet or a blanket, each part of the body being exposed as required, and then covered again. The face and head are first bathed with cold water, after which the attendant begins with the right arm, and proceeds over the body in the usual order.

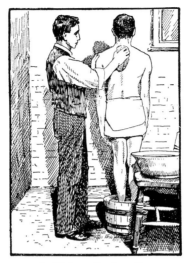

(Fig. 122) Tepid or Cold Sponge Bath

The strength of the tonic will depend upon the temperature of the water and the amount of moisture in the mitten, also the amount of friction employed.

Hysteria, neurasthenia, anaemia, chlorosis, consumption, diabetes, rickets, dyspepsia, scurvy, paralysis agitans, and other chronic wasting diseases are benefited by the cold mitten friction. It is a good general preventative against colds and influenza.

The Tepid or Cold Towel Rub (50° to 90° Fahr.).

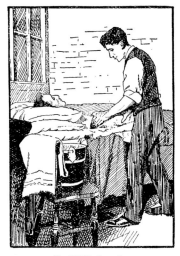

(Fig. 123) Wet Towel Rub

The higher temperatures are for feeble patients. First bathe the face and neck with cold water, and then apply a cold compress to the head.

The patient may lie or stand, as circumstances demand. Wring a linen towel rather dry from the cold water and lay it on the patient's chest, then rub the towel briskly, not the skin. Much of the success of this treatment depends on the rapidity and vigour of the friction. The patient's skin should be left in a healthy glow *(Fig. 123)*.

This is a stronger tonic than the cold sponge, and is not always suitable for weak and infirm patients, especially if they do not react readily.

The Salt Glow.

Soak some common salt in water for a few moments and rub the moist salt upon the surface of the body. The patient may lie on a marble slab, or stand in a foot tub of hot water. Begin with the right arm, then the left arm, the chest (gently), the abdomen, back and finally the legs and feet.

The Oil Rub.

This delightful measure is generally useful in almost all conditions of health and disease. Olive oil, coconut butter, or some other lubricant may be used. But little oil is required, and this should be rubbed well into the skin. Any surplus oil may be removed by a towel.

Moderate friction should be used, this being at once a mild tonic, and to a certain extent, a sedative. It is a fallacy to think that the body is nourished to any considerable extent as a result of the inunction. Under the most favourable conditions, only the merest trace of oil enters the circulation.

The oil rub is a good finishing treatment after a warm bath and a salt glow, or following cold mitten friction. It may be given to advantage under almost any conditions, and forms by itself a good mild tonic.

The Internal Use of Water

Next to oxygen, water is the most indispensable of all the bodily requirements, and life would cease to exist sooner if deprived of water than of food. All of the living cells of the human body are literally bathed in water continually.

"Water-drinking is an internal bath; it dilutes the fluids of the body in which the cells and fibres are bathed; it purifies the body by diluting the medium in which it lives. By the free use of water, the movement of the mass of liquid in which the living elements of the human body perform their work is quickened, and the stream of life runs clear and pure." *

Physiological Effects of Water-Drinking.

Water taken internally exerts a direct stimulating effect upon the kidneys, the glands of the skin, and, indeed, upon all the excretory organs. It encourages both the constructive and the disintegtrative processes of the tissues, serving as the medium for carrying food material to, and removing waste from, the tissues.

*Dr. J.H. Kellogg, in "Rational Hydrotherapy"

Cold Water Drinking.

Under ordinary conditions, cold water, that is water at a temperature of between 60°to 70°Fahr., is the proper drink, and may be considered to be a true tonic. Very cold water is often helpful in fevers and to treat certain other conditions, but it should be taken slowly and in small quantities.

Free water-drinking is desirable for all persons, but it is especially valuable in various pathological conditions, particularly in all rheumatic and gouty disorders. Obesity, diabetes, gall-stone colic, chronic indigestion, biliousness, constipation, alcoholism, among other more or less chronic disorders, are all greatly benefited by the free use of water.

A pint of cold water at night and another an hour before breakfast, make one of the most effectual remedies for chronic constipation. Free water-drinking is also a successful measure in combating colds.

For fevers, a patient may have all the water he wants. Dr. Kellogg recommends a glass each hour. It is a great aid in the elimination of poisonous wastes from the body.

Avoid cold water, except in small quantities, when wearied or sweating vigorously.

Hot Water Drinking.

It is remarkable to note the very high temperature at which water and other fluids are often taken. Extremely hot drinks cannot fail to be injurious if taken habitually. Even hot water (120°to 140°Fahr.) soon has a debilitating effect upon the body, and it is not wise to persist in its daily use, unless prescribed by a physician. Acidity of the stomach can usually be relieved by drinking a glass of hot water. Gastralgia, or stomach-ache, is also relieved by the same measure.

Lukewarm water, taken very freely, makes a simple and very efficient emetic. One or two pints are necessary as a rule. The addition of a little mustard makes the emetic still more effectual.

How Much to Drink.

There are two extremes. Most people do not drink enough, some scarcely taking water at all. A few others might be considered disciples of Priessnitz, who frequently recommended ten, fifteen, or even twenty pints per diem. Of course this is altogether too much, and can scarcely fail to do damage. We would recommend drinking between two and five pints per day, according to the nature of the diet, climate, and other circumstances.

When to Drink.

The question, when ought one to drink, is briefly answered by replying: any time except at meals. Sufferers of indigestion ought to wait one or two hours before taking any considerable quantity of water.

The objections to drinking at meals are as follows:-
1. It interferes with thorough mastication of the food.
2. It dilutes the saliva and gastric juice.
3. It destroys the delicate flavours of food.
4. It retards both salivary and peptic digestion.

Mineral Waters.

It has been well said that "mineral waters are simply diluted drugs," and this is absolutely true. The best water is the purest. There is, however, no objection to aerated distilled water, which is absorbed into the system sooner than plain water.

Hard water should be boiled, the longer the better. Boiling precipitates some of the salts. Those living in chalky districts would do well to use distilled water, which is easily prepared by a simple family still, to be had at small cost. Such temperance drinks as home-made lemonade, orangeade and other juices diluted with water are both wholesome and refreshing.

The Enema or Water Injection.

The enema consists of an injection of water or of specially prepared fluids into the rectum and colon by means of a bulb or fountain syringe. The quantity varies, but usually amounts to from one to four pints. A larger quantity is likely to produce permanent dilatation of a weak colon, and the use of three or four quarts, or even more, at one time, is a reprehensible practice.

Among the more common varieties of enemata are the following:-

Plain enemata.	Tannic acid enemata.
Soap enemata.	Graduated enemata.
Starch enemata.	Nutrient enemata.

In giving an enema, have the patient lie on the left side, or on the back with hips elevated. To get the fluid into the deeper recesses of the colon, put the patient in the knee-chest position, resting on his knees and chest.

The Plain Enema.

The best all-round temperature is 80°Fahr. At this temperature water has a tonic effect on the bowels. If warm, the effect is relaxing. A cold enema of 60° to 70°Fahr. reduces fevers, has tonic effects on the colon, and stimulates peristalsis. Only a half to a pint of cold water should be given if it is to be retained.

Soap, Starch, and Acid Enemata.

Soap-Suds, made from a good quality grade of soap, will more quickly and thoroughly relieve the bowels than will plain water. The temperature should be between 70°and 80° Fahr.

The starch enema is very soothing, and is helpful in relieving diarrhoea. It is prepared by making a very thin paste of starch and water. Usually only one or two pints are injected.

A teaspoonful of tannic acid to one pint of water is the proportion ordinarily used for acid enemata. Other acids and antiseptics are occasionally employed.

Graduated and Nutrient Enemata.

For those who have acquired the enema habit, the graduated enema affords a simple means of getting rid of it. Begin with three pints at 90°Fahr., and reduce the quantity one quarter of a pint and two degrees daily. In chronic cases, it is often necessary to repeat the treatment, and even then it fails at times.

Nutrient enemata, as the name indicates, contain nourishment and are very useful for feeding patients who are unable to take food by the stomach. A well-beaten, raw egg in plain or peptonised milk makes a very good combination. Before injecting the nutrient it is necessary to wash out the bowel by giving a full plain water enema. Such enemata should be given under the direction of the family physician.

INDEX